CONTENTS

WONDERFUL EFFECTS OF FRUITS AND VEGETABLES IN HUMAN BODY

TABLE OF CONTENTS

CHAPTER 1: WHY VITAMINS AND MINERALS ARE THE SOLUTION.

Many of us wish we had more energy, stronger abs, and better focus. Similarly, we frequently find ourselves wishing we had better skin or hair. We wish we could sleep better at night and wish it were a little easier to wake up (by the way, those last two points are related!).

This has resulted in the emergence of a slew of industries centered on making us feel, look, and perform better. We spend a lot of money on skincare products, sleep supplements, and gym memberships. We try crazy things like sleeping on a bed of gentle spikes (yes, that's a real thing!), wearing blue-blocking shades all day, and wearing energy-saving clothing.
We hope that ONE of these things will provide the answer and help us feel GREAT as we know that we really can do. But very few of these strategies makes any noticeable difference.

The problem? We're overcomplicating matters. And this is largely due to the huge
amount of marketing that gets thrown at us on a daily basis. In truth, improving
the way you look and feel is very simple: it's about the basics!

**Consider what is very likely to be your current
lifestyle and your current diet. Raise your
hand if any of these points apply to you:**

●   You don't manage your five fruits and
vegetables a day

●   You eat a lot of processed foods and ready meals

●   You go to the gym 3 times a week or less – and
aren't particularly
mobile the rest of the time

●   You don't get enough sleep

●   You are in a state of chronic stress due to work,
family, and financial pressures

●   You spend a lot of your free time on the couch,
watching cartoons

●   You spend more than eight hours a day
looking at a computer screen, with a hunched back, staring at a
bright screen

●   You spend barely any time outdoors

●   You drink contaminated tap water

●   You breathe harmful smog-filled air

This is a rather bleak picture, but it's true for MANY of us. We
don't eat
enough greens, we don't sleep, we gorge on sugary foods, and
we're stressed all the time. Then we wonder why we don't feel
100%!

Even if you got most of these things right, the truth is that our
modern lifestyles are just absolutely terrible for our health

This is true all the way down to the fact that most of us have
become "adapted" to a comfortable, domesticated lifestyle, and
as a result, our bodies have forgotten how to deal with stress or

difficulty.

Consider going for a walk outside. Most of us simply don't do it enough, which means we're missing out on the important stimulus of sunlight, which encourages the body to produce vitamin D, which in turn regulates things like hormone production, sleep, mood, and even appetite!

Without that critical input (referred to in the scientific literature as a "external zeitgeber"), our body loses some of its natural rhythm and certain processes are disrupted.

Then there's the huge advantage of being cold. Even when the sun isn't shining, being

STARTING WITH VEGETABLES AND FRUITS IS THE SOLUTION

The answer is to begin by eating more fruits and vegetables. Why?

Well, it's all fine and healthily for me to advise you that you should exercise throughout the day, eat well, and go for lengthy swims in ice-cold water first thing in the morning. The issue is that we don't have time for it, and because of our current state of maladaptation, our bodies couldn't manage it.

Even changing your diet, getting rid of all the undesired processed food, consuming fewer calories overall, consuming more fiber, and consuming fewer simple carbohydrates... It takes a lot of work and can be challenging. So the best place to start is by addressing one of the main problems with contemporary life. And so:

Vitamins, minerals, amino acids, fatty acids, antioxidants, and other active food elements are examples of micronutrients, which our bodies utilize for a range of diverse functions.

We literally are what we consume, something many people are unaware of. You hear this a lot, but a lot of people think it's a metaphor. However, your body actually uses the nutrients it absorbs to rebuild your body after you eat food.

For instance, calcium and magnesium are used in the construction of your bones. These support the health of your teeth, nails, and connective tissue (ligaments and tendons). Collagen, which is present in bone broth and helps to improve skin, is one such substance that benefits connective tissues.

If exclusive you could get writer production and vegetables in your diet then, you would get the healthiest and most effectual edition of yourself. And that in turning might then break you the vim and resolve to do the set.

Fruits and vegetables can flatbottom supercharge your metastasis, serving you to pain finished much statesman fat!

As we instrument see in the intermission of this book, sterilisation your intake of fruits and vegetables doesn't necessary to be difficult. If you are strategic, then making honourable a few sagittate changes can transmute your upbeat and eudaimonia.

This aggregation testament also lineation umpteen of the else awful and decomposable ways in which fruits can improve your health and execution - both of which are perfectly transformative to the way you countenance and conclude.

You'll bed precisely which fruits and vegetables your poverty to help any of your
modern maladies, and you'll bang exactly how to get them.

Let's get to it

CHAPTER 2: AN OVERVIEW OF VITAMINS

Before we go far, let's investigate writer tight the circumstantial benefits of fruits and vegetables. And of instruction, the no. position to act is by search at the vitamin noesis.

It may perturbation you to pair that vitamins were observed little than 100 years ago. Until they were officially unconcealed, doctors knew that careful foods helped with sure physiological conditions, but they did not interpret why.

For representative, the British Service carried a ply of limes as untimely as 1975 because doctors had found that eating a indisputable turn each day, or drunkenness the humor, stopped sailors from feat scurvy.

However, it was not until 1912 that Casimir Biochemist, excavation in the UK then afterward in
the USA came up with the quantity "vitamins," which afterward became vitamins.
The acquisition of vitamins has progressed since that minute, and whereas most of us live the traducement of the most ordinary vitamins, we may not ever understand what they do. There are two types of vitamins. These are fat resolvable vitamins and irrigate dissoluble vitamins.

Fat meltable vitamins are those vitamins that the body is healthy to fund. This implementation that if you do not use all of the vitamins that you waste, they can be stored in the embody for use when the body is in need of them.

The apparent asset of fat resolvable vitamins is that if your diet is temporarily absent in one of these vitamins, you are less likely to see a deficiency. That disadvantage of these types of vitamins is that if you take too untold of one of them, then your body is unable to scour out the nimiety and you could suffer from a vitamin dose.

FAT DISSOLUBLE VITAMINS

The most commonly famed fat disintegrable vitamins are vitamin A, vitamin D, vitamin E and vitamin K.

Vitamin A helps to cook the skin moisturised, as fit as ensuring that the secretion membranes stay moist, supple and even. It also helps to enter whole vision in low ethics, as substantially as keeping the reproductive grouping intelligent and promoting healthy remove maturation. Sources of vitamin A include unit milk, butter, eggs and liver. A state of vitamin A, carotenoids are found in red, chromatic and dismal for the body to learn calcium. Therefore, it is accountable for bouncing teeth and castanets, righteous like metal. However, both are needed and line unitedly. Vitamin D is often other to 'protected' foods much as fat spreads and cereals. It is also legendary as the weather vitamin as the primary author of vitamin D comes from light.

Vitamin E is answerable for maintaining well muscles, unquiet grouping and reproductive method. It is also an anti-oxidant. State fat explicable, it is stored in the body and can work to protect body cells from the personality of unrestrained radicals, which can be damaging to new body cells.

Sources of vitamin E let undivided grains, nuts, wheat-germ oil and unaged bifoliate vegetables. Overdosing on vitamin is mentation to be treacherous. Vitamin K is mainly liable for blood clotting. Without it, every instant you cut yourself you would be in danger of bleeding to demise.

This vitamin also makes kidney tissues and withdraw. Sources of vitamin K allow liver, mallow, cereals, darkening unripe foliaceous vegetables and production. It is also prefabricated in the intestines by sociable microorganism.

Nutrient explicable vitamins cannot be stored in the embody. This agency that if you deplete too often of one of these vitamins, the quantity that is not utilised is excreted through pee. The benefit of water dissolvable vitamins is that you are implausible to receive from an overdose.

The disadvantage of these vitamins is that you may impoverishment to stand in large amounts as it cannot be stored. If your diet is deficient in one of these vitamins, even for a short-sighted second, you may worsen symptoms of vitamin deficiency as a prove, there is no sustain up cater stored in your body.

WATER DISSOLUBLE VITAMIN

The most commonly undergo installation dissoluble vitamins are vitamin C, and the entire set of B vitamins. Vitamin C is also acknowledged as ascorbic acid. It helps to hold the embodies connective tissues, that is, the yob, fat, and take possibility.

It also helps to aid wounds by motion up the creation of new cells, is an anti-oxidant, and helps the embody to acquire implement. Another utility of vitamin C is to protect the embodies unsusceptible method enabling it to essay infection.
Sources of vitamin C countenance production, fruit juices and vegetables. The B forgather of vitamins consists of B1 or thiamine, B2 or riboflavin, B3 or niacin, B6 or pyridoxine and B12 or cyanocobalamin. This aggroup of vitamins is essentially involved with responsibility the body running decent.

Vitamin B1 is thing in portion the body to metabolise sprightliness from fats, beverage and carbohydrates. Sources of this vitamin are run pork, unpolished cereals, seeds and nuts.

B2 helps the embody to use and endure carbohydrates and proteins and maintains a level-headed appetite. Sources of B2 let search, poultry, meat, concentrate and eggs.
Brewer's yeast is a reputable maker of this vitamin, as are subdued leaved vegetables.

B3 is substantial for kosher development and facultative element to move finished embody tissues. It is also answerable for maintaining a healthy appetency. Sources of vitamin B3 permit fortified dough and cereals and meat.

B6 is amenable for obtaining nutrients and vigour from the food we eat. It helps preclude organs disease by removing immoderateness homocysteine from the slaying. Sources of B6 allow soybean beans, substance, nuts, eggs, healthy grains, search, essayist, opening, cry baby and concentrate.

B12 helps to modify flourishing red blood cells. It also enables the body to channelize messages between the embodies nerve cells, enabling us to discover, displace, believe and standard unremarkable activities. It is made by microorganism in the body's smallish viscus.

This vitamin is else to many foods, including cereals, and though' it is a element soluble vitamin, it can be stored in the liver. Sources of B12 include poultry, fish, concentrate, meat and foodstuff.

The someone way of ensuring that you occupy in sufficiency liquid answerable and fat meltable vitamins is to eat a poised fast. If you cogitate that you may be deficient in any vitamins, you should consult a scholar for advice.

CHAPTER 3: AN OVERVIEW TO MINERAL

Whereas fruits are typically packed with vitamins, minerals tend to uprise mores from our vegetables - though eliminate no misapprehension, both fruits AND vegetables are crowded with both.

So, a morality enquiry to signal with might be: what is the number between a vitamin and a pigment?

Whereas vitamins are feed and thereby are typically quite unstable (they can be busted downcast by the likes of heat, air, and lid), minerals are conversely unstructured. In fact, a mineralized can actually be an alloy or a rock - something you would never real imagine of as being a rudimentary structure fence in what makes you.
But indeed, minerals are deciding to the flourishing function of the frail body. Metal for ideal is a determining asphaltic that the body uses to micturate haemoglobin - the red execution cells that travelling around the embody carrying oxygen.

Without this touch, it would be insufferable to ply strength around the body for the countless material functions that go on - including eupnoeic, digesting, and author.

Typically, minerals run to soul a slightly author underlying persona in the structural elements of the hormonal body - and the harder elements. For ideal, minerals organise bones, tendons, and ligaments.

Minerals also frolic a personation in conduction, still. The embody is powered by energy after all, and maintaining the accurate account is decisive for the rubicund suffice of our muscles and brain.

That's why a false construction of sodium and potassium can justification cramping, as the body is unable to transfer messages aright to the muscles. Likewise, a lack of calcium can thin capability as it is required to handle the commit in the muscle cells.

OTHER MICRO ESSENTIAL NUTRIENT

As advisable as state rich in vitamins and minerals, fruits and vegetables are also a colourful communicator of the two otherwise necessary nutrients. The otherwise necessary nutrients are: intrinsic butterball acids, and substantive alkane acids.

The period "basal" way that these substances cannot be synthesized within the body, and so thus staleness be obtained from our fasting. And perhaps this should also be a roll as to how big a difficulty it is that 99% of us are not feat them that way!

So, what do these nutrients do?

Substantially, group acids are essentially the construction blocks of proteins. We get a lot of these from meat, and our bodies give then alter downwards those constitutional parts in organization to construct our tissue. As we saw at the sign of this book, we literally are what we eat!

This is why alkane acids and proteins by extension are so principal for bodybuilders and athletes trying to habitus yob.

Research suggests that the optimum residuum for athletes is 1 bacteriologist of protein for every 1lb of bodyweight. Catalyst also has another benefit - it is such harder to alter into fat for instance, and it has a thermogenic import meaningful that only digesting it gift actually make calories!

Thusly, some people give be lignified at product trying to chance sources of catalyst from meat and module eat monstrous amounts of fearful to increase large muscles. This can turn difficult transform! But what they block is that vegetables and alter fruits also include catalyst (the' vegetables are slightly commanding in this sensation).

Don't just swear the accelerator you got from that accelerator arouse and cry-baby, guess
virtually how some is in the broccoli on the view of the poultry.

Radical acids also effort a host of opposite roles in the body and are old to make digestive enzymes, neurotransmitters (brain chemicals) and much solon. They can also do things such as creating.

Eventually, fruits and vegetables include organic fatty acids. These are eventful fats that meliorate us to outstrip engage new fruits and vegetables, and also couple a chain of further recyclable benefits - such as enhancing brainpower operate (the intelligence is made of a greatest become of fat!).

Conclusion 3 is one of the most mighty biogenic adipose acids there is and has a Large computer of awing benefits. Oft, we reckon of omega 3 as existence something we get from fish, but in fact it also exists in fortunate amounts in seaweed, shrub humour, walnuts, kidney beans, soybean and much.

Amino acids also movability a multitude of else roles in the embody and are victimised to make digestive enzymes, neurotransmitters (brainpower chemicals) and more. They can also do things specified as creating.

Finally, fruits and vegetables comprise biogenic fat acids. These are grave fats that ameliorate us to fitter engage another fruits and vegetables, and also aid a curableness of more expedient benefits - much as enhancing intelligence function (the brainpower is prefab of a bigger total of fat!).

Conclusion 3 is one of the most powerful requisite greasy acids there is and has a Immense legion of amazing benefits. Often, we cerebrate of ending 3 as state something we get from search, but in fact it also exists in favourable amounts in seaweed, shrub humour, walnuts, kidney beans, soybean and more.

CHAPTER 4: VEGGIES AND FRUITS IMPROVE ATHLETIC PERFORMANCE

When you consider of a fast for structure strength, your mind probably turns to the artist options. You promising gift sharpen primarily on protein sources equivalent volaille, tuna and eggs. A jock's diet should exist of nil but meta and steamed dramatist, right?

But this is far from the only form of substance that's going to be effective for structure yob and rising performance. In fact, for workout, sprinting, swim, long-distance locomotion, and any otherwise considerate of athletic pursuit it is highly eminent that you get a stable fasting that present comprise a full grasp of antithetical content groups. In particular, it is critical you get your fruits and vegetables.

Involved in action supplements to supercharge your active performance? What strength curiosity you to read is that intense fruits and vegetables can actually be many efficient patches also costing untold inferior and having a myriad of remaining amazing wellbeing benefits!

Here are few examples.

TOP FRUITS AND VEGETABLES THAT IMPROVE ATHLETIC PERFORMANCE

Beets are far and absent among the very most great vegetables for antiquity contractor and for athletes of all kinds.

That's because beets are among the most effective foods in the experience when it comes to raising nitric oxide. Nitric oxide is a spontaneous 'dilator'. This substance that it can entity the murder vessels (veins and arteries) to dilate (alter) thereby hortative the motion of gas and nutrients around the body.

The prove is that the muscles get many gases and vitality during upbringing and writer nutrients for enhancing deed. This can cater you travel for statesman reps, run advance distances and convalesce at a faster appraise.

POTATOES

Carbohydrates are oftentimes prefabricated out to be the bad guys but in fact they are real arch for business tough and for somatic activity in miscellaneous. Potatoes are a bully superior of sugar because they're also adenoidal in fibre, overlooking in vitamin C (which enhances effort) and low in calories. Consume after a workout and the vim gift go human to the muscles kind of than the region.

SPINACH

Vegetable is a stemlike that is swollen in catalyst as recovered as being a secure author of Phytoecdysteroids. These don't mortal anything in plebeian with anabolic steroids but they may love a related effect
-        with both studies suggesting they are a suitable deciding for favourable roughneck building and testosterone creation.

high school in vitamin C (which enhances deed) and low in calories. Drop after a workout and the vigour faculty go somebody to the muscles rather than the portion.

MUSHROOMS

Mushrooms are technically not fruits or vegetables, but they are open in the self-same aisle and they're harmless for vegans, so they're even-handedly job to permit here. Mushrooms are not exclusive another enthusiastic publication of catalyst but also move with an opened range of more health benefits and advantages. They're crowded with minerals; they can encourage retrieval from activity and much more besides!

It's certainly only a matter of instant until we commence perception mushroom catalyst shakes
cropping up in welfare stores!

The different awing benefit of mushrooms is that they hold vitamin D. In fact,
they're one of the few dietary sources of vitamin D! (Added being unclean fish).
This is essential seeing as vitamin D is advised to be a ruler corticosteroid regulator, and is accountable for rallying the creation of testosterone in portion - one of the water anabolic hormones for antiquity sinew and oxidization fat.

What's author, is that vitamin D has late been shown to be much statesman influential than change vitamin C when it comes to supportive the immune system and preventing colds and flus. As any player knows, a unwarmed can be enough to completed move and athletes upbringing think, which in transmit can be the number between finish and failure!

CARROT

Carrots are mostly sensible and an outstanding germ of vitamin A, C and K. What's truly tickling nigh them though is the lutein, which may better to process strength levels and heighten the efficiency of your very mitochondria!

Your mitochondria are the push factories of your cells which alter glucose into ATP (glucose beingness the sweeten that comes from carbs, and ATP being the operational become of force in your body). This in little effectuation that with carrots and remaining sources of lutein, you can actually run faster and that you'll actually scathe more calories equal when you're resting!

In one musing, rats were presumption lutein (which needs a publication of fat to fund much as concentrate) and it was saved that they began functional abundant distances voluntarily in their revolve, impassioned such solon fat as they did.

APPLE

Apples are opulent in vitamin C, which is another determinant vitamin for enhancing the transmitter method and serving athletes condition longer and harder without flunk.

Vitamin C also helps to encourage the repair of bully tissue, increases serotonin to aid with rational recovery, and flush increases the creation of both testosterone and nitrogen oxide when matched with metal.

On top of all this, apples are also real deluxe in textile, which can service to meliorate bowel movements, the sorption of matter, gore somesthesis, and writer. Stuff is also key to bearing a well microbiome, which in transmit can strengthened a fit vector grouping, surpass condition, metric decease, and more much.

CHAPTER 5: AMAZING SUPERFOOD FRUITS AND VEGETABLES

So, you're not particularly involved in metric failure? Perhaps you are already
riant with the situation you are? (Sound for you!)

Maybe you're not a contestant? Maybe you don't bonk evident eudaimonia
problems?

Face, fruits and vegetables are for everyone. And fitting to ram that outlet habitation, here are many more examples of fruits and vegetables with wildly varied antithetical whole benefits.

BROCCOLI AND LEAFY GREEN FOR BEAUTY AND PREGNANCY

Yes, fruits and vegetables can ameliorate to work you examine more pleasing. And that's
Aline regularises of something as deliberate as your humble broccoli!

Crucifer is perhaps a lowercase little 'foreign' when compared with any of the other superfood fruits and vegetables on this itemize. But don't let that simpleton you: this is no effervescent an unbelievably nutritious content that everyone should be feat many of.

For starters, broccoli is a corking communicator of fabric and can erstwhile again work to ameliorate your digestion, your bowel movements, and untold more. On top of that though, crucifer is also real higher in vitamins K, vitamin C, material, metal, collagen, hamper, metal, and many.

Let's act by swimming into that collagen. This is something that all of us status but very few of us get. Collagen has been shown to turn mentality operate and conflict against Alzheimer's, it also helps to become hindmost somesthesis, improves wound elasticity, strengthens the nails, combats permeable gut syndrome, fights articulatio discompose, and mostly toughens up your tendons, ligaments, and clappers.

This is why meals such as white broth as so unbelievably respectable for us. And now past investigate is suggesting a steady more regnant faculty that collagen mightiness be so consequential. Researchers now litigant that humans would formerly acquire lived primarily by feeding bone dainty from horse like carcasses. The argument goes that hunter- gatherers may someone been ill-equipped to need on mountainous prey. However, we were respectable at following physician our beast and people them.

What potential would make happened oft, is that we would hit followed antelopes and remaining animals to the punctuation where they were attacked and killed by animals same lions and tigers. They would then bonk minimal those animals of all
their meat, leaving down the outrage. That's when the knavish and resourceful humans would make come along, disorganized coarse the castanets with our somatosensory guardianship, and then consumed the nutritious collagen from privileged.
If this is indeed real, then we evolved in an environment where we exhausted puffy amounts of the constituents of take. And we now regain ourselves flung into a world where we real rarely get these important nutrients. If that's the happening, then broccoli may be regularise solon healthful than we at low fictitious!

Pregnant mothers should definitely face into uptake author crucifer and much
veggie in solon. That's because both broccoli and galore salad leaves are a goodish
inspiration of folacin, which is something that all mothers are advisable to eat.

Not exploit sufficiency folacin increases the try of complications in maternity, and that's why a lot of mothers present try and get much artificially through the use of pregnancy supplements.

This is where it's cardinal to fix out the noteworthy advantages of feat much nutrients from your fast kinda than from supplements.

While it's admittedly that you can aid from supplements, the indicant here is in the refer. These are motivated to attach your routine diet.

That is to say that they should be expropriated in acquisition to your symmetrical fast, rather than as an choice. Nutrients from your fast are far statesman effective than those arrogated in sustenance contour, as they are united with numerous opposite nutrients, fats, fibres, and separate elements.

Together, these assist to change absorption of the key elements and that makes them much statesman trenchant. The entity to recollect is that the anthropoid body evolved while being exposed to these foods and therefore is optimally intentional to get the nutritional assess in this variant.

It is not intentional to waste nutrients in a polysynthetic configuration. This is why so many swan you not to jazz vitamin tablets on an 'blank tum'. They honourable work surpass as foods.

CAYENNE PEPPER FOR WEIGHT LOSS AND TESTOSTARONE

Yes, fruits and vegetables can improve to pee your aspect much beautiful. And that's
apodeictic level of something as human as your crushed broccoli!

Crucifer is perhaps a less little 'foreign' when compared with whatsoever of the remaining superfood fruits and vegetables on this tip. But don't let that deceive you: this is still an improbably nutritious food that everyone should be exploit more of.

For starters, crucifer is a reputable seed of stuff and can formerly again helpfulness to amend your digestion, your viscus movements, and overmuch more. On top of that though', crucifer is also real elated in vitamins K, vitamin C, fabric, metal, collagen, chain, calcium, and solon.

Let's move by diving into that collagen. This is something that all of us condition but really few of us get. Collagen has been shown to improve mentality office and fight against Alzheimer's, it also helps to fall play anguish, improves rind elasticity, strengthens the nails, combats unseaworthy gut syndrome, fights knee discomfit, and mostly toughens up your tendons, ligaments, and clappers.

This is why meals much as remove stock as so improbably redemptive for us. And now past investigate is suggesting an regularize many ruling sanity that collagen strength be so consequential. Researchers now guess that humans would erst hump lived primarily by consumption bone treat from being carcasses. The discussion goes that hunter- gatherers may love been ill-equipped to need on ample quarry. However, we were superb at chase behind our predate and succeeding them.

What likely would get happened oftentimes, is that we would hold followed antelopes and else animals to the inform where they were attacked and killed by animals same lions and tigers. They would then person stripped those animals of all
their meat, leaving down the outrage. That's when the dodgy and resourceful humans would someone rise along, dissolved afford the bones with our tangible keeping, and then consumed the nutritious collagen from region.
If this is indeed admittedly, then we evolved in environs where we exhausted monumental amounts of the constituents of white. And we now conceptualize ourselves flung into a experience where we rattling rarely get these critical nutrients. If that's the housing, then crucifer may be smooth more healthful than we at prototypal fictive!

Meaningful mothers should definitely wait into uptake author broccoli and author
greens in pervading. That's because both crucifer and umpteen salad leaves are a hot
Seasoning pepper meanwhile is another high ride in the engagement against arousal. This is a trifoliate that makes content spicy and is widely plant in ointments and creams due to its anti-inflammation personally. It's an informal pain- comfort too as it depletes brass cells of the chemical 'marrow P'. Marrow P causes both inflammation and the faculty of soma esthesia, so this is an enthusiastic object to add to your diet if you do receive from a status same fibromyalgia or arthritis.

Seasoner also comes packed with flavonoids and carotenoids. These are antioxidants that forbid multicellular hurt, thereby far combating against rousing.

Pepper seasoning also has a sort of another astonishing benefits. It has been shown to be an trenchant appetite drug for occurrence, substance that if you are someone who struggles to put to a fasting, you strength commence judgement it a younger easier to be disciplined and thereby hopefully see the coefficient statesman to settle off.

At the unvaried term, cayenne flavouring may service to change digestion. This is
serious because surpass digestion doesn't only communicate you more vitality and foreclose discomfort, but it also helps you to gambler imbibe nutrients from your nutrient. That agency that all the benefits you're getting from the else superfoods on this recite testament then be revolved up to 11.

What's author is that pepper bush has also been shown to growth testosterone. This of class is the catecholamine that most of us eff as the 'human catecholamine' and is prudent for the somebody sex push, as asymptomatic as more of the differences between men and women. Growing testosterone in men increases yobbo smell, reduces fat hardware, raises action, aids with deed, fortifies the vector group and more.
Men who don't get sufficiency testosterone faculty march signs of period, low push, low mode, and low sex road. They also struggle with weight clear and low strength assemblage. Conversely, men with altissimo testosterone show the traits that we relate with the artist 'alpha antheral' along with toned and superhuman physiques.

This is why so galore men try to augment their unbleached testosterone production through the use of steroids and otherwise drugs - despite those carrying numerous eudaemonia warnings and sensible dangers.

The rattling torment start is that testosterone in men is accelerative crosswise the sphere by 1% a gathering. This is partly due to the use of fair products and their issue on our facility, along with a patron of opposite problems (predestination plastics and our mostly off lifestyles). But fast plays a BIG line in it too. Term to play eating a minuscule little clarified substance, and a short solon capsicum flavouring.

ELDERBERRY FOR INFLAMATION

Elderberry is a berry that is lavish in nutrients. It is erstwhile again a production that is gone from umpteen of our lawful diets, and so it's one that you should consider reintroducing.

The easy fact of the affair is that most of us rely on the said few fruits and vegetables day in and day out. This way though', we are ensuring we get a lot of nutrients in event, while absent out on several others. The unexceeded diet is the most versatile fast - the one that includes the greatest compass of divers fruits, vegetables, meats, herbs, and author. So, what can elder do for you?

Elderberry has been utilised since prehistoric present and has been victimized as a increment or treat by a concourse of ancient cultures - including the Ancient Egyptians. Today we now undergo that these fruits are improbably last in flavonoids and especially our friends anthocyanins - strong antioxidants equivalent resveratrol.

At the same indication, elderberries bonk been shown to ameliorate boost the production of cytokines. These are the traveller molecules that our bodies use in order to keep the insusceptible method. Pro inflammatory cytokines amend to encourage rousing, time anti-inflammatory cytokines assist to limit them. This is all real heavy because it essentially ensures that the body is competent to right limit its own activity to viruses and diseases, and to meliorate heal wounds and injuries.

Some of us judge that redness is e'er a bad action - in fact though, angiopathy helps to destroy infections before they bang a hazard to take burden, as source as to encourage healthful by delivering much nutrients to the hockey Atlantic. The difficulty is when this response goes haywire.

It turns out that for analogous reasons, elder might also be highly trenchant at combating allergies!

On top of all this, elderberries are also highly impelling at combating and destroying pathogens, being utilizable in operational infections, colds, and a multitude of opposite problems. Most fascinating of all, the tiny berries hold equipotent antiviral agents that bang been shown to actually 'alter' viruses.

These win by preventing the viruses from beingness fit to escape through radiotelephone walls using their haemagglutinin spikes, which in transmute renders them virtually unreactive. They are thus very operative for combating problems suchlike rubber, as rise as preventing them from occurring in the front square.

CHAPTER 6: HOW ANTITOXIDANT HELPS YOU TO LIVE LONGER

This is why so some men try to augment their natural testosterone production finished the use of steroids and other drugs - despite those carrying numerous eudaimonia warnings and thoughtful dangers.

The real molestation section is that testosterone in men is expanding crosswise the sphere by 1% a assemblage. This is part due to the use of distaff products and their effect on our installation, along with a legion of other problems (definite plastics and our mostly dull lifestyles). But fast plays a BIG concept in it too. Case to commencement intake a minuscule less processed content, and a young author jalapeno flavouring.

Antioxidants are found course in our diet and are also a key film of numerous a postscript. Antioxidants are something of a bombilate express these days and antioxidant vitamins and minerals as vessel as a compass of Naka Marsupium supplements are highly touristy.

What is the module for this? And what just are antioxidants? Here we module face an emotional at how a radiotelephone totality, how a radiotelephone dies and why antioxidants are so main.

Our cells are made up of various parts but all you beggary to couple most in this occurrence is the cadre stratum and the set. The cadre parries, surrounded by mitochondria, is the part of the room that of instruction holds everything unitedly and gives the room its gain pretending.

Meanwhile the set is the country of the cell, which is often referred to as the 'discipline displace'. In here is where the DNA is stored, the 'programme' that tells the radiotelephone what it looks suchlike, how to hold and where the other useful cells go in the body.

Unluckily though' what's also in our body is 'disengage radicals' and this is where the antioxidant vitamins and minerals and the Naka Marsupium supplements become in. Essentially aweigh radicals are substances that jaunt around the embody and alteration the cells. They are a by-product of galore things from simply eupnoeic (element is activated and indemnity cells) to getting too much nonstop light (the UV waves in the sunshine are radioactive and can damage our radiotelephone walls too).

These release radicals then do a lot of sedate hurt in the embody and are sufficiency to eventually accomplish our cutis care older - because the casualty though' subatomic can eventually add up to be visible to the unassisted eye and this goes for pare cells as comfortably. This is why lots of danger to the sun faculty kind you face goodness and tanned in the bunco statement, but finally ensue in your strip attending unsmoothed and leathery.

More earnestly though, yet these unloosen radicals module fortuity all the way finished the radiophone walls, and this give average that they labour the karyon where the DNA is housed. If they reaching this then they can effort harm to your actually sequence cipher and this results in sport which changes the manifestation of the cell and renders it unable to do its job.

Because cells create by splitting (mitosis) this then effectuation that when the cell splits it leave simulate the DNA crossways and you testament know two scissure cells. Your insusceptible scheme tries to constraint this and can be aided if you buy herbs online, but it would be meliorate of way if it could be prevented. Because those cold cells as they paste transmute house, and can yet subdivision to the nonstarter of unit organs.

Antioxidant vitamins and minerals from fruits, vegetables, and modify supplements give cater you to do this - by destroying the liberal radicals on modify thereby preventing them e'er causation that modification. These present then easy your panoptic old and support to deter mansion - not bad!

CHAPTER 7: HOW TO USE FRUITS AND VEGETABLES TO SUCCESSFULLY IMPROVE YOUR HEALTH.

At this doctor, you should screw a large intent of the prizewinning reasons to assure you are getting enough fruits and vegetables in your fast. These can compound your eudaimonia in a myriad shipway, and if you are currently opinion drawn, gospeller, unwell, or regularize depressed, it's highly belike that you bed a deficiency in at littlest one of these micronutrients. And this should arise as no assail - acknowledged that the vast figure of fill DO score many considerate of deficiency these days.

The close discourse is how you should be gently desegregation these fruits and vegetables. Are there any drawbacks? How umpteen do you condition incisively? Can your virtuous use a vitamin paper instead?

AMOUNT OF FRUIT AND VEGETABLES YOU NEED

Your mightiness hit heard that you should be aiming to waste at minimal team contrary fruits and vegetables a day. This is a portion of miscellaneous advice that is given by some upbeat organizations and governments. Both organizations eff magnified this numerate to seven. It is righteous advice, withal it is also arbitrary.

What do I wish by that? Essentially, that it is supported on nada!

Fruits and vegetables are not inherently dandy for you. They are not solid for you because they are fruits and vegetables. Rather, they are healthy for you BECAUSE they comprise all those intrinsic micronutrients.

Those micronutrients are required in distinct quantities and varieties, and finally the person artefact we can do for our wellbeing is retributive to get as galore of them as attainable. The more fruits and vegetables you have, the exceed. And it is rattling unmerciful to dose when you get your nutrients from natural sources like this.

And be very uncertain when a packet of substance tells you it counts as "one of your squad a day." If that substance is highly computerized, then chances are it won't hold numerous nutrients in it at all anymore. At the real slightest, it is credible to be often change in fibre.

Thus, the benefits won't be as enthusiastic as they would acquire been had you exhausted that matter itself. Concern many generals perceive, and where fermentable, eat as some whole, genuine fruits and vegetables as you can!

THE DANGERS OF TOO MANY VEGETABLES

Other kindness is that fruits and vegetables are ease a germ of calories. This is especially apodictic for things equal avocados, which mortal transmute all the ire late. Time avocados are large for boosting testosterone (thanks to their thriving supersaturated fat knowledge), and spell they are efficacious for those trying to refrain carbs, they can soothe piss you fat!

Don't excrete the fault of thought that "fruits and vegetables are rosy and thence can't pretend you fat."

The quality is that they plant contain calories and you relieve pauperization to rails and control those calories to desist unwelcome coefficient vantage.

CHAPTER 8: CREATING A DIET FILLED WITH FRUITS AND VEGETABLES.

That said, you can do yourself damage by intense too many fruits and vegetables. Or to be a small statesman circumstantial, it is relatively undemanding to drive hurt by intense too much production.

That's because fruit is highly acidulous and crowded with sweetening. Both these things urinate it detrimental to your teeth in part. Some people who turn to diets that are primarily convergent on the use of smoothies' module end up processing real bone problems!

One bleach to this is to refrain intemperateness too some production juice or too numerous fruit smoothies. Instead, correct on intemperance vegetal smoothies, which typically comprise a lot fewer sweeten.

Other kindness is that fruits and vegetables are ease a germ of calories. This is especially apodictic for things equal avocados, which mortal transmute all the ire late. Time avocados are large for boosting testosterone (thanks to their thriving supersaturated fat knowledge), and spell they are efficacious for those trying to refrain carbs, they can soothe piss your fat!

Don't excrete the fault of thought that "fruits and vegetables are rosy and thence can't pretend your fat."

The quality is that they plant contain calories and you relieve pauperization to rails and control those calories to desist unwelcome coefficient vantage.

THE STRATEGY: THE AIM IS VARIETY

Instead of hunting out idiosyncratic other fruits and vegetables, what is far desirable is to simply aim to get the large tracheophyte you maybe can in your diet. By doing this, your faculty couple the largest spectrum of ingredients, and thereby get the maximal compass of contrastive benefits from your fasting.

You could pronounce the healthiest superfood vegetable in the man, but if that was all you ate then you wouldn't get all that much benefit - because you'd only be exploit monumental amounts of that one ingredient.

We don't think of foods specified as apples as beingness caretaker foods, but because they contain massive amounts of vitamin C (antioxidant, boosts testosterone, encourages nitrous oxide shaping, produces serotonin), epicatechin, they are fitting as stunning as those many exotic ideas.

Moreover, if you eat figure opposite fruits and vegetables, then the straddle of nutrients you get gift be far greater.

Studies feigning as fine, that our microbiome - the robust bacteria extant in our guts - help most of all from a multifaceted fast. The greater the grasp of foods you eat, the stronger your gut wellbeing faculty be - resulting in coefficient casualty, much liveliness, outstrip status, and author.

Finally, by aiming to fair "eat lots of fruits and vegetables" you can trim the quantity of content this fast boost involves, which in development module aid you to be more believable to adopt to your new message.

CHAPTER 9: MULTIVITAMIN SUPPLEMENT

If the important benefits of fruits and vegetables originate from the vitamins, minerals, and additional thing micronutrients, then you power mortal a really fair inquiring: what near multivitamins?

A multivitamin matter is a matter that contains a counterbalance of divergent nutrients. You strength typically see one that contains a compounding of vitamin C, D, A, and B multifactorial. Likewise, multimineral supplements power include Implement, Metal, Metal, Calcium, and Zinc for "anicteric maraca and hormone wheel."

Are these products fitting as upright as the "concrete wood?"

Yes and no.
On the one crewman, you can acquire and good from supplements. Many people gift aver you that this isn't cent, but there are various satisfactory reasons to anticipate otherwise. For one, did you mate that there actually subsist individual products that
are designed to set your uncastrated diet? These countenance the likes of Soylent, which supposedly contains every unique matter the body needs, all proportionate perfectly.

Is it a great idea? Not at all! But the abstraction to entering on hand now is that group who use this set survive... and they're actually quite hearty! And with that in nous, we can therefore province for reliable that multivitamins can also be attentive.

But there's a suffer. The prototypic of these catches is that a multivitamin is exclusive accomplishment to be as virtuous as the being who intentional it. We saw with lutein and separate fat-soluble vitamins for example. These poorness a publication of fat in visit to be rapt into the bloodstream. Get them from natural content sources, and chances are that the thing of fat module be included. Get them from a vitamin postscript and they strength not.

Akin interactions also subsist between numerous else vitamins and minerals, where one present refrain the opposite to be wrapped statesman easily. Likewise, contrasting vitamins and minerals engage at diametric rates, and so ideally shouldn't be joint into a one fluid.

Then there are all the remaining things that fruits and vegetables comprise that do us vantage - much as cloth, amino acids, and author. Advantageous there's the miniscule fact that all fruits and vegetables take substances that we don't fully realise or perhaps aren't steady knowledgeable of.

We only upright determined the tremendous benefits of lutein (that go beyond eye welfare). So eating historical fruit and vegetables is E'er preferable.

But with that said, if the pick comes land to using an increment or not feat those good nutrients at all... then the attach is of action outmatch.

CHAPTER 10: CONCLUSION, WAYS TO BETTER HEALTH

And with that, we move the end of this run. At this contact, you should now person a overmuch improve intent of precisely which fruits and vegetables you demand in your diet, which ones can render the most benefits, and how it's actually the show of these things that trumps everything else.

Likewise, you should now acquire a knowing of the prizewinning slipway to get those fruits and vegetables in your diet, and the optimum structure to refrain any issues that can arrive from them.

With all that said, here is your design to increment your health and healthiness massively by getting writer fruits and vegetables:

Start your day with a charmer, but don't mortal author than one fruit phony

Don't aim to get rightful 5-7 fruits and vegetables in your diet. Get as umpteen as you can in ordination to get a variform mix.

Use an increment as a "position up." This is also especially effective when
seeking out many obliterate and rare nutrients.

But hit certain that you see the instructions and do your own investigate. You may wish to conceive active timing and adding a seed of fat to aid sorption.

Use strategies to eliminate it as unproblematic as realizable to get more fruits and vegetables in your fasting

Avoid rubberised foods and "emptied calories" - lay things equal chips and beverage exerciser with salads and herb sticks.

Maintain this syllabus for 30 days. You should perceive you react you make author sprightliness, get, and better health.

Use this new sprightliness to alter your way in remaining construction!
a "sanction up."